CANCER AND MODERN SCIENCE™

TESTICULAR CANCER

Current and Emerging Trends in Detection and Treatment

HEATHER HASAN

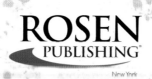

ROSEN
PUBLISHING®

New York

To Joseph: I have really enjoyed getting to know you over the years.
Please know that you are tremendously loved.

Published in 2012 by The Rosen Publishing Group, Inc.
29 East 21st Street, New York, NY 10010

Library of Congress Cataloging-in-Publication Data

Hasan, Heather.
Testicular cancer: current and emerging trends in detection and treatment / Heather Hasan.—1st ed.
      p. cm.—(Cancer and modern science)
Includes bibliographical references and index.
ISBN 978-1-4488-1312-4 (library binding)
1. Testis Cancer—Popular works. I. Title.
RC280.T4H37 2012
616.99'463—dc22

2010013022

Manufactured in the United States of America

CPSIA Compliance Information: Batch #S11YA: For further information, contact Rosen Publishing, New York, New York, at 1-800-237-9932.

On the cover: By using a special electron microscope, researchers were able to photograph these three fast-growing testicular cancer cells. The teratoma cancer cells have large, irregular nuclei (pale brown) and green cytoplasm.

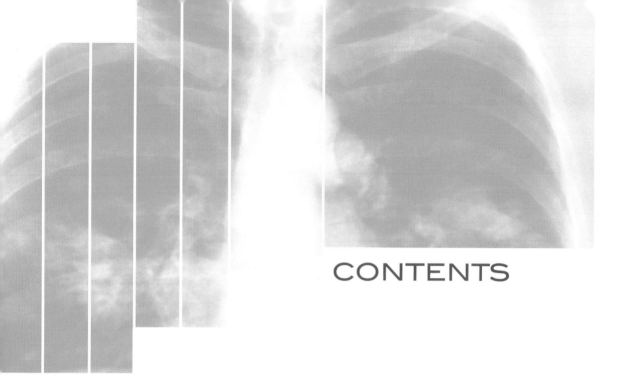

CONTENTS

INTRODUCTION

Doctors during ancient times knew that cancer usually returned, even after it was physically removed with surgery. Nearly two thousand years ago, Aulus Cornelius Celsus (25 BCE–50 CE), a Roman who is believed to have been a physician, wrote eight books about medicine (*De medicina octo libri*). In one of these books, he reported, "After excision, even when a scar has formed, none the less [sic] the disease has returned, and caused death." This grim view, that cancer cannot be cured, has persisted in some ways, even until today. It is true that only about forty years ago, a diagnosis of testicular cancer was virtually a death sentence. In 1970, 90 percent of men with testicular cancer died of the disease. However, testicular cancer is now a success story in the field of cancer medicine.

In 1965, Dr. Barnett Rosenberg, a professor of biophysics and chemistry at Michigan State University in East Lansing, became interested in the phenomenon of cell division. He decided to experiment with how electricity would affect the division of cells. Rosenberg used a type of reaction called electrolysis, a method that passes current through a substance, resulting in many kinds of chemical reactions. Usually with

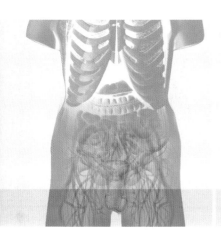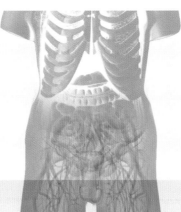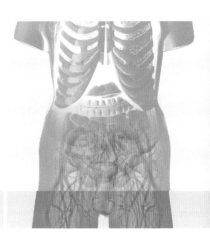

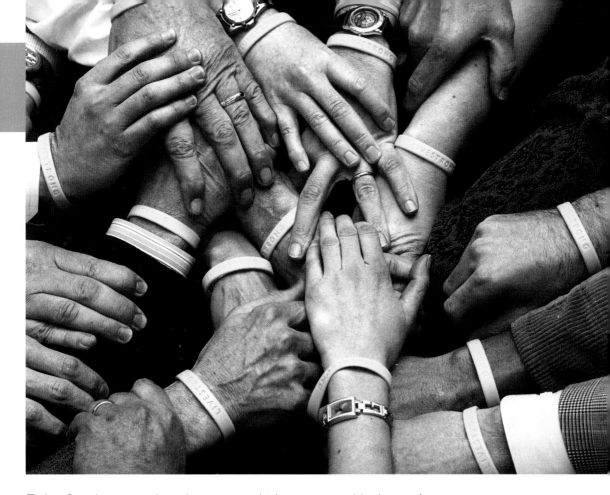

Today, foundations such as Livestrong, which was started by Lance Armstrong in 1997, raise testicular cancer awareness and money to fight the disease. Livestrong supporters wear yellow bracelets to show their encouragement.

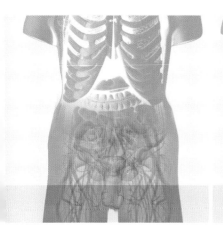
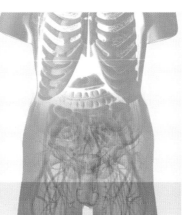
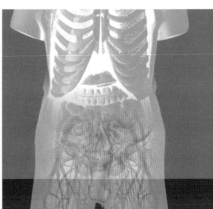

electrolysis, electrodes are placed on either end of a container of solution. An electrical current is then passed through the solution from electrode to electrode. Rosenberg placed a solution containing the cells of *E. coli* bacteria in a container with platinum electrodes on either side. When he turned on the electric current, he was surprised to see that the bacteria cells had stopped dividing! As Rosenberg worked to understand this mystery, he realized that a chemical reaction was responsible for the change. After much study, he determined that the electricity had prompted a reaction between the platinum electrodes and some of the nutrients from the bacteria solution. The reaction had produced a compound called cis-diamminedichloroplatinum (II). Rosenberg reasoned that if this compound could stop cell division, it might be a useful anti-cancer drug. Cisplatin, as he called it, underwent some drug testing and was approved for use as a cancer drug in 1978.

This unintentional discovery of cisplatin has revolutionized the treatment of testicular and other cancers. In the 1970s, only about 10 percent of the men who were diagnosed with testicular cancer survived the disease. Today, this disease has a survival rate of more than 95 percent! People such as Lance Armstrong, one of the world's best cyclists, are living testimonies to the vast improvements in testicular cancer treatment. By the time Armstrong sought help for his testicular cancer in 1996 (three years after he noticed a lump in one of his testes), it had already spread to his lungs, abdomen, and brain. Years ago, there would have been no hope for this world-champion cyclist. However, through modern advances, Armstrong was treated successfully. He not only recovered but also went on to win the Tour de France seven years in a row! Testicular cancer is often completely curable, especially if it is found and treated early. Nevertheless, fear of a cancer diagnosis and lack of knowledge about the disease still keep some men from seeking help until it is too late. The goal of this book is to educate people about testicular cancer, its types and risk factors, and its diagnosis and treatment options.

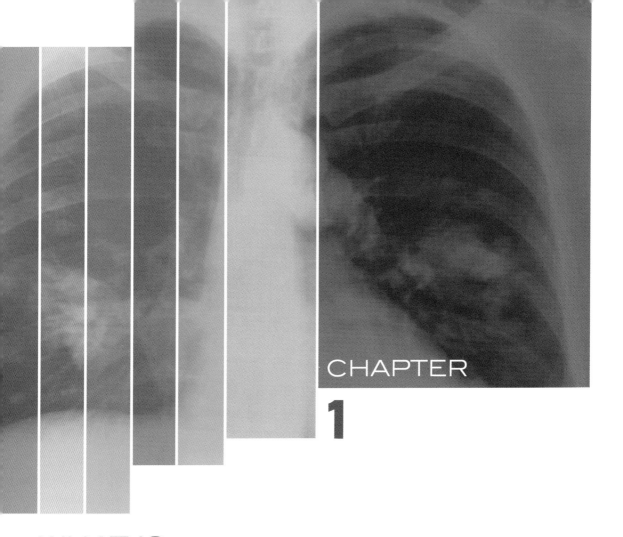

WHAT IS TESTICULAR CANCER?

Cells are the building blocks of life. They are the smallest units of living organisms. In fact, the human body is made up of billions of cells that are so small, they can only be seen with a microscope. When cells work together to do a specific job, they are called tissues. In the same way, tissues that work together to perform a task form organs.

Normal, healthy cells grow and divide in a planned, organized way. When they are damaged or old, they repair themselves or die. This process keeps the body in good condition. Sometimes, though, cells lose the ability to limit and direct their growth. These damaged cells are called cancer cells. Unlike healthy cells, cancer cells just continue to grow, divide, and multiply without order. They don't even die when they are supposed to. Cancer cells usually clump together to form excess tissue called tumors. Tumors damage the normal, healthy cells and tissues around them. This damage can make a person very sick. Testicular cancer occurs when cells in one or both testes become abnormal and begin to grow uncontrollably. The testicles are an important part of the male reproductive and endocrine systems.

The Male Reproductive and Endocrine Systems

The organs of the body are organized into different groups called organ systems. All of the organs in a system work together to perform a specific task. One important organ system is the reproductive system. The male reproductive system consists of the organs that males need to reproduce, or create new individuals.

The male reproductive organs work together to produce, nourish, and transport sperm into the reproductive system of a female during sexual intercourse. Sperm is the male reproductive cell. It fertilizes the female's egg to create an embryo and thereby begin pregnancy. The male reproductive organs, or genitalia, are located both inside and outside the pelvis. This location of the reproductive organs is unlike that in females, whose reproductive organs are located entirely within the pelvis. Outside the pelvis, males have a pouch of skin called the scrotum. The scrotum hangs beneath the base of the penis. The word "scrotum" comes from the Latin word scroutum, which means "leather pouch for arrows." The testicles, or testes, are located inside the scrotum. The testicles are two oval-shaped organs, each of which is somewhat smaller than a golf ball, about 2 inches (5 centimeters) long and 1 inch (3 cm) wide. These organs are responsible for producing and storing sperm

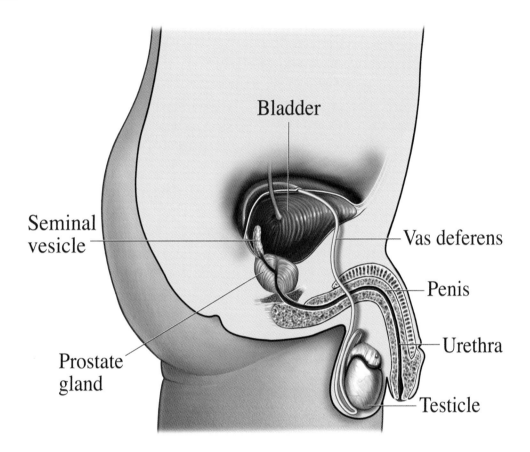

Bladder

Seminal
vesicle

Vas deferens

Penis

Urethra

Prostate
gland

Testicle

The organs of the male reproductive system are shown here. The testicles lie outside the body because sperm production requires a temperature that is three to five degrees below body temperature. However, if it becomes too cool on the outside, the scrotum will contract to bring the testes closer to the body for warmth.

In addition to the testicles, other important organs and structures of the male reproductive system include: a duct system through which the sperm passes to reach the outside of the body; the accessory glands, which produce fluid to lubricate the duct system and nourish the sperm; and the penis. Sperm that is produced in the testes is carried through two small tubes (vas deferens) to the seminal vesicles. In the seminal vesicles, fluid from the prostate gland is added. The fluid travels through the tube at the center of the penis called the urethra. Both urine and sperm pass through the urethra but at different times.

The testicles are also part of the endocrine system. The endocrine system is made up of glands, which are organs (such as the testes) that secrete chemicals to keep the body working properly. These chemicals are called hormones. One of the hormones produced by the testes is testosterone. Testosterone is important in a male's body. It is the hormone that causes males to grow taller, speak with a deeper voice, develop bigger muscles, grow body and facial hair, develop a larger penis and testicles, and produce sperm.

Types of Tumors

There are two basic types of tumors: benign and malignant. Some lumps of tissue in the body do not grow in an unlimited, aggressive manner, and they do not spread to other parts of the body. These tumors are called benign tumors. They are not cancers. Benign tumors can be harmful to a person's health if they grow large and push against a vital organ, such as the brain. However, these tumors can usually be removed by surgery, and they are not likely to return. Most benign tumors are harmless. In fact, the word "benign" means "gentle" or "mild." Some tumors of the testes are benign, but most are malignant.

Malignant tumor cells invade and destroy nearby, healthy tissues. Unlike benign tumor cells, they may travel through the lymph and

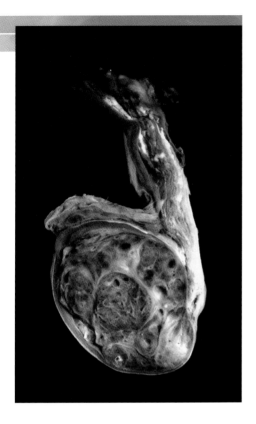

This photograph shows a cross section of a testicle that contains a teratoma, a type of malignant tumor.

blood vessels to other parts of the body. Lymph is a colorless body fluid containing white blood cells. It is transported throughout the body in a way that is similar to how blood vessels transport blood. Malignant cancer cells travel through the body, starting new tumors in other areas. This process is called metastasis. When a cancer spreads in this way, it is said to have metastasized. Death occurs from cancer when the spreading cannot be stopped. The cancerous cells take the place of healthy cells. This process causes organ systems to fail, and the body cannot function properly. Cancer cells may spread to other organs, but the cancer type is still the same as the original growth. For example, if cancer were to start in the testes and then spread to the lungs, it would still be considered testicular cancer. When it spreads, testicular cancer most often spreads to the lymph nodes, abdomen, lungs, retroperitoneal area (the area in the back of the abdomen), and spine.

TYPES OF TESTICULAR CANCER

The testicles contain many different kinds of cells. Each of these can develop into one or more types of cancer. The most common type of cancer occurring in the testes is germ cell tumor. This type of cancer develops within the germ cells. The word "germ" means "seed." The germ cells are the cells that produce sperm in males. According to the American Cancer Society, nearly nine out of ten testicular cancers begin in the germ cells. There are two main types of germ cell tumors in men: seminomas and nonseminomas. According to the Testicular Cancer Resource Center, about 40 percent of germ cell tumors are pure seminomas.

AN EARLY RECORD OF CANCER

The Greek physician Hippocrates (about 460–377 BCE) gave cancer its name. He called it *karkinos*, a word that was used to describe a crab. Hippocrates thought cancer looked like a crab. Cancer was known long before Hippocrates named it, however. The oldest recorded case of cancer was written on papyrus in Egypt in 1500 BCE. The ancient document described eight cases of breast cancer. The ancient Egyptians attempted to treat this cancer by using a hot instrument they called "the fire drill" to cauterize it. The papyrus also gave evidence that the ancient Egyptians understood the difference between malignant and benign tumors. The Egyptians also described how they surgically removed cancers on the skin's surface. This procedure was similar to that used by doctors today.

Seminomas are organized into two main subgroups: classical and spermatocytic. By far, the most common form of seminoma is classical seminoma. It accounts for more than 95 percent of seminomas. This type of cancer usually occurs in men who are in their late thirties to early fifties. Spermatocytic seminomas are rare and tend to occur in older men. The average age of men affected by this type of cancer is fifty-five. These tumors grow more slowly and are less likely to spread to other areas of the body than classical seminomas. In general, seminomas respond better to treatment than do nonseminomas.

Nonseminoma subtypes represent the remaining 60 percent of germ cell tumors. This type of tumor most often occurs in men in their late teens to early forties. They grow fast and spread quickly. There are four types of nonseminomas: embryonal carcinomas, teratomas, yolk sac tumors, and choriocarcinomas. Embryonal and teratomas are the most common forms of nonseminoma. According to the American Academy of Family Physicians, they each account for approximately 26 percent of the cases of testicular cancer. Embryonal carcinoma is highly malignant and aggressive. It grows rapidly and tends to spread to the lungs and liver. Teratomas are made from the types of cells found in an embryo. Because the cells in an embryo can become any kind of tissue, it is not uncommon for them to contain hair or teeth! Fittingly, teratoma means "monstrous cancer." Teratomas are usually benign and localized (mature teratomas) but are sometimes made up of more immature cells with potential to spread throughout the body (immature teratomas). Very rarely, teratomas can have malignant transformation. Yolk sac tumors and choriocarcinomas are both very rare types of testicular cancer. They each account for only about 1 percent of testicular cancers, according to the American Academy of Family Physicians. Though rare, yolk sac tumors are the most common type of tumor that affects children under the age of three. Choriocarcinoma is very

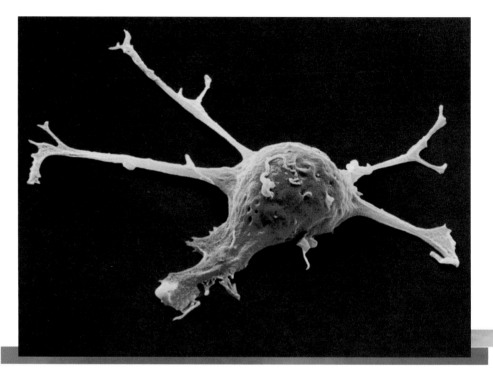

This cancer cell (with cytoplasmic projections) has been magnified and color-enhanced.

aggressive, often spreading quickly to the lungs. It also often does not respond well to treatment. Most nonseminoma tumors are made of a mixture of two or more types of testicular cancer. A treatment plan for such tumors is usually designed against the most aggressive type so that the cancer is not undertreated. For instance, a nonseminoma testicular cancer that has both teratoma and choriocarcinoma parts should be treated as a choriocarcinoma. Similarly, a testicular cancer that has seminoma and nonseminoma components should be treated with nonseminoma therapy.

Another type of testicular cancer is called stromal cell tumor. This type of cancer only accounts for 3 to 4 percent of all testicular cancers, but it represents 20 percent of childhood testicular tumors. This type of cancer develops in the supportive tissue and hormone-producing tissue, or the stroma, of the testes. Stromal cell tumors are often benign and do not spread beyond the testes. They can usually be cured with surgical removal. A few stromal cell tumors do metastasize, however. These cancers have a poor outlook because they typically do not respond well to treatment. The two main types of stromal cell tumors are Leydig cell tumors and Sertoli cell tumors. Leydig cell tumors form from normal Leydig cells, the cells in the testicles that produce testosterone. Sertoli cell tumors develop from normal Sertoli cells in the testes. The Sertoli cells support and nourish the sperm-producing germ cells.

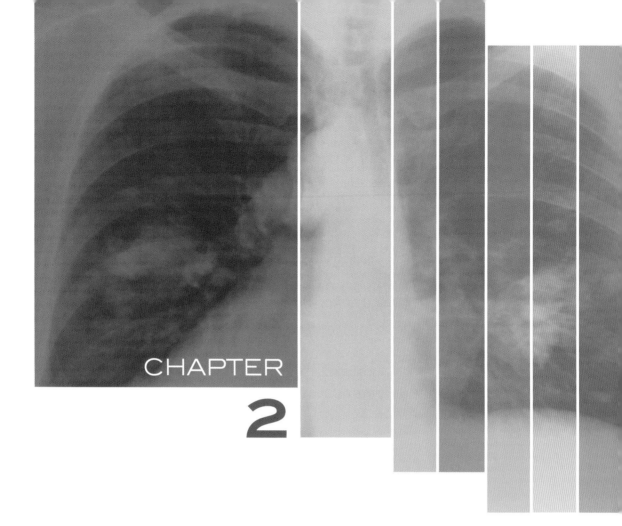

WHO IS AT RISK?

According to the American Cancer Society, about eight thousand men are diagnosed with testicular cancer each year. The exact cause of testicular cancer is not known. It is not always clear why one person gets it and another does not. Nevertheless, scientists have identified certain risk factors for developing testicular cancer. A risk factor is anything that increases a person's chance of developing a certain disease.

Every disease has different risk factors. For example, people who smoke are at a higher risk than nonsmokers for developing lung cancer.

Even so, the fact that a person has risk factors for a certain disease does not mean that he or she will develop that disease. Sometimes, a person with many risk factors for a disease will not develop it, whereas someone with no risk factors will. Some risk factors, such as smoking, can be controlled. Others, such as a person's race or age, cannot be changed.

Knowing the risk factors can help people make informed decisions about their behavior. If individuals have many of the risk factors for a certain disease, they can be monitored by health professionals for signs of it. Some of the risk factors for testicular cancer are age, race, cryptorchidism (a condition in which one or both testicles fail to descend normally), and a personal or family history of testicular cancer. However, people who develop testicular cancer often have no known risk factors. Meanwhile, the number of men who are developing the disease is increasing. Research is still being done to identify other causes of testicular cancer.

AGE AND RACE

More than 70 percent of cancers affect people who are older than sixty. For this reason, most people think of it as a disease of the elderly. Yet, there are some cancers that are more likely to affect young people. Testicular cancer is most frequently detected among younger men. It usually affects men between the ages of twenty and twenty-nine, and it is the most common form of cancer in men between the ages of fifteen and thirty-five, according to the National Cancer Institute. It is important to remember, though, that testicular cancer can affect males of any age. Although testicular cancer is more common among young men, it is a fairly rare disease. The chance of a man developing testicular cancer in his lifetime is only about one in three hundred, according to the American Cancer Society.

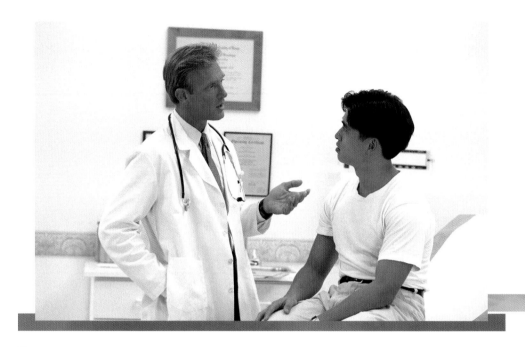

There is no way to prevent testicular cancer. However, it is very treatable if it is found early. Doctors should check a man's testicles during his annual physical exam.

Race is another factor in the development of testicular cancer. Testicular cancer is more common in Caucasian men than in men of other races. It is especially common in Caucasians who are of northern European descent. The incidence of men developing testicular cancer is highest among those living in the United States and Europe and lowest among men living in Asia and Africa. According to the American Cancer Society, white Americans in the United States are more than three times as likely to get testicular cancer as Asian American and Native American men and have about five times the risk of African American men. The risk for Hispanics falls somewhere between that of Asian Americans and non-Hispanic whites. The reason for this difference is not currently known.

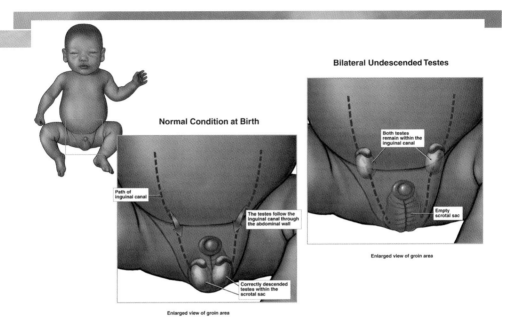

Bilateral Undescended Testes

Both testes
remain within the
inguinal canal

Empty
scrotal sac

Enlarged view of groin area

Normal Condition at Birth

Path of
inguinal canal

The testes follow the
inguinal canal through
the abdominal wall

Correctly descended
testes within the
scrotal sac

Enlarged view of groin area

Here, the testes of a male infant (top left) *are shown first in the normal position* (center) *and then in the undescended position* (right).

CRYPTORCHIDISM

A congenital abnormality is a defect that is present at birth. Research has shown that males born with abnormalities of the penis, testes, or kidneys have an increased chance of developing testicular cancer. One congenital abnormality that has been linked to testicular cancer is cryptorchidism, or undescended testes. As a baby boy grows inside his mother's womb, his testes form inside his abdomen. Normally, the testes move down, or descend, into the scrotum before birth. In some cases, however, a baby is born with an undescended testis. Though cryptorchidism does not cause testicular cancer, it is one of the main risk factors for developing the disease. According to the American Academy

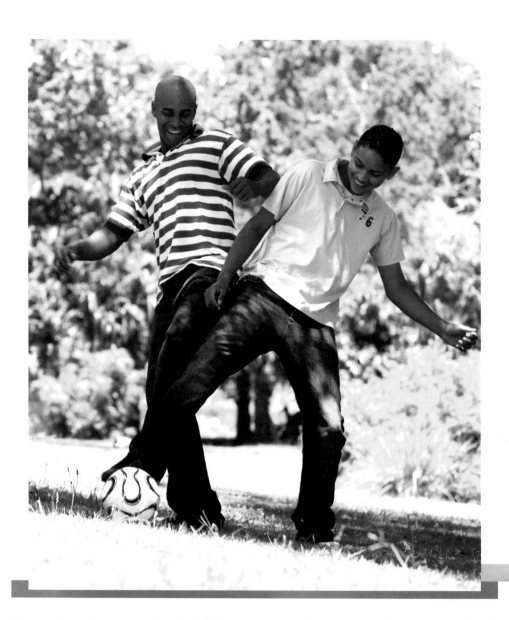

Researchers have recently identified some genes that seem to be associated with testicular cancer. These findings may make it clearer why sons of fathers who have had testicular cancer have an increased risk of developing the disease.

of Family Physicians, one in ten cases of testicular cancer occur in men who have had cryptorchidism.

In about half of the babies born with cryptorchidism, the testis descends on its own by the time the baby is six months old. In some cases, however, the testis must be surgically moved into the scrotum to preserve future fertility (the ability to reproduce). Ordinarily, this surgery, which is called orchiopexy, is performed if the testicle has not fully descended by the time a boy is a year old. The increased risk of later testicular cancer development remains even after the condition has been corrected with surgery.

PERSONAL AND FAMILY HISTORY

A personal history of testicular cancer is another risk factor. If a man has previously had testicular cancer, he is at an increased risk of getting it again. Studies have shown that 3 to 4 percent of men who have had testicular cancer in one testicle will eventually develop cancer in the other testicle. The risk for a man to develop testicular cancer is also greater if family members have had the disease. According to studies done at the Institute of Cancer Research, a man is eight to ten times more likely to develop testicular cancer if he has a brother with the disease and about four times as likely if his father has had it than someone with no family history of testicular cancer.

MYTHS AND FACTS

MYTH Strenuous physical activity can cause testicular cancer.

FACT Most studies have not found that strenuous physical activity can increase the chance of getting testicular cancer. In fact, physical activity has been linked to a lower risk in several other forms of cancer.

MYTH Injury to the scrotum can cause testicular cancer.

FACT Some patients with testicular cancer do have a history of scrotal injury. However, many doctors think that the injury just calls attention to a tumor that was already there.

MYTH Testicular cancer is contagious.

FACT Although some people in the seventeenth and eighteenth centuries believed that cancer could be spread from person to person, it cannot.

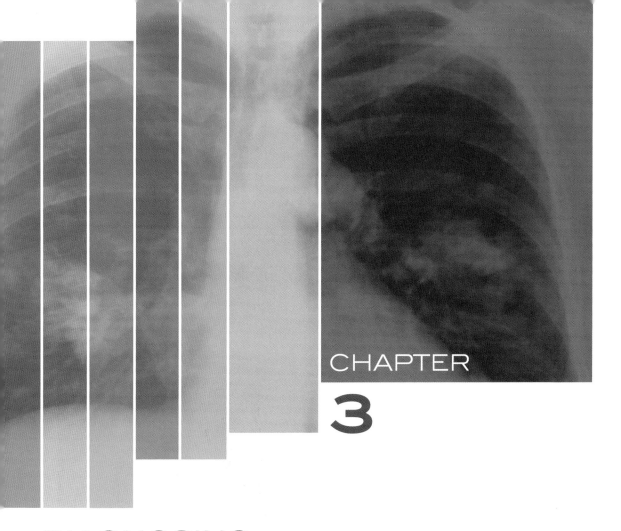

DIAGNOSING TESTICULAR CANCER

Even though testicular cancer is most common in young men, the disease does occur in other age groups, too. Therefore, all men should be aware of its symptoms. One of the most common symptoms of testicular cancer is the swelling of the testis. Another very common symptom is a pea-sized lump on the testis. Other symptoms include hardening of the testis, a dull ache in the lower abdomen or in the groin, a feeling of unusual heaviness in the scrotum, a sudden buildup of fluid in the scrotum, tiredness, and an overall feeling of being unwell. A man may

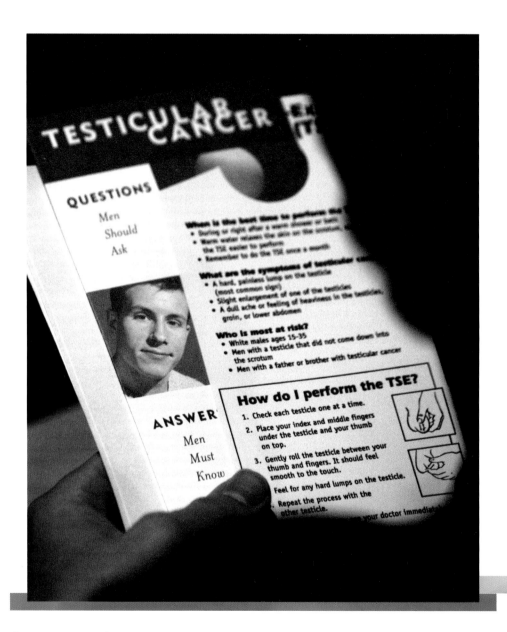

Because testicular cancer is more common among younger men, it is important for teenage boys to learn how to perform a testicular self-exam.

also have pain or discomfort in the testis or scrotum. This pain may come and go. More severe symptoms include back pain, breast tenderness, shortness of breath, and coughing up blood.

TESTICULAR SELF-EXAMINATION

Many times, men first discover testicular cancer themselves. They may notice a hardening of the testis, a change in the size of the testis, the presence of a lump, or pain in the testis. Sometimes, testicular cancer is found by accident. Other times, it is found by doing a testicular self-exam (TSE). A TSE takes about three minutes to perform. It should be done standing naked in front of a full-length mirror. If one leg is elevated, it is easier to get a better view of the scrotum. During the exam, a man should look for any swelling on the skin of the scrotum. He should also examine each testicle with both hands, feeling for any lumps. Often, a lump found at an early stage may only be the size of a pea and will most likely be painless. The best time to perform a TSE is after a warm bath or shower, which allows the scrotum to relax and makes it easier to locate lumps.

Men who examine themselves regularly become familiar with the way their testicles normally feel. It is then easier for them to notice a change. Some health professionals recommend that men between the ages of fifteen and forty do testicular self-exams on a monthly basis. However, many do not believe that it is necessary for TSEs to be done that often. A monthly TSE, however, is recommended for men who are at high risk for developing testicular cancer, such as those who have had cryptorchidism or those who have a personal or family history of testicular cancer. In any case, a man should always see a health professional if he thinks there might be a problem. He should not wait for the symptoms to go away by themselves. Testicular cancer is almost always curable if it is found early.

WHEN IT IS NOT TESTICULAR CANCER

The presence of swelling, pain, or a lump may not necessarily mean that a man has cancer. These symptoms may be the result of things such as injury or infection. Orchitis (inflammation of the testis) and epididymitis (inflammation of the duct system called the epididymis) can both cause pain and swelling. These are usually caused by viral or bacterial infections, some of which are considered sexually transmitted diseases. Any bacterial epididymitis is generally treated with antibiotics. Pain in the testes may also be caused by testicular torsion. With this condition, the spermatic cord (the cord from which the testis hangs) becomes twisted and can choke off the blood supply to the testis. Any extreme pain in the testis should immediately be evaluated by a doctor, as testicular torsion can result in a dead testis in a matter of hours. Another condition, called spermatocele, results in the formation of a cyst in the epididymis. The cyst is usually filled with a milky fluid that contains sperm. Spermatoceles may or may not be painful.

VISITING THE DOCTOR

Most health professionals believe that it is a good idea to routinely visit a doctor for a physical or wellness visit. This allows doctors to screen for different diseases and conditions and offer the patient advice on how to remain healthy. During a physical exam, the health professional will examine the patient from head to toe, including the groin and genitalia (the penis, scrotum, and testes). The doctor will palpate, or touch, the organs, feeling and looking for swelling, lumps, or the shrinking of the testes (called testicular atrophy). One of the first steps in establishing a diagnosis of testicular cancer is making a detailed medical review. A doctor will examine a patient's past health, his family medical history, his testicular cancer risk factors, and his symptoms. If testicular cancer is suspected, a doctor will then arrange for some tests. Some common tests that are used to help diagnose testicular cancer are blood tests and scrotal ultrasounds. If these tests are worrisome, a testis biopsy or an orchiectomy is performed to obtain tissue to examine under the microscope. These tests will help the doctor determine the type of cancer and the best treatment for the patient.

BLOOD TESTS

One of the first tests a doctor performs on a patient who might have testicular cancer is a blood test. Though there is not yet a single blood test that can confirm the presence or absence of cancer, a blood test can help guide a doctor's diagnosis. Substances called tumor markers are given off by cancer cells and can be detected in the blood. The presence of certain tumor markers may indicate testicular cancer. There are three tumor markers used to detect various forms of testicular cancer. Alpha-fetoprotein (AFP) is a protein that is produced by a baby as it develops in the mother's womb. It is not found in adult men but is produced in high amounts by some nonseminomas, particularly yolk sac tumors. Beta human chorionic gonadotropin (β-hCG) is a hormone that is normally found in the blood of pregnant women. A high amount of β-hCG in the blood in males is worrisome for nonseminomatous (and occasionally, seminomatous) germ cell tumors. The third kind of tumor marker that can indicate the presence of testicular cancer is lactate dehydrogenase (LDH). LDH is an enzyme that is found in many

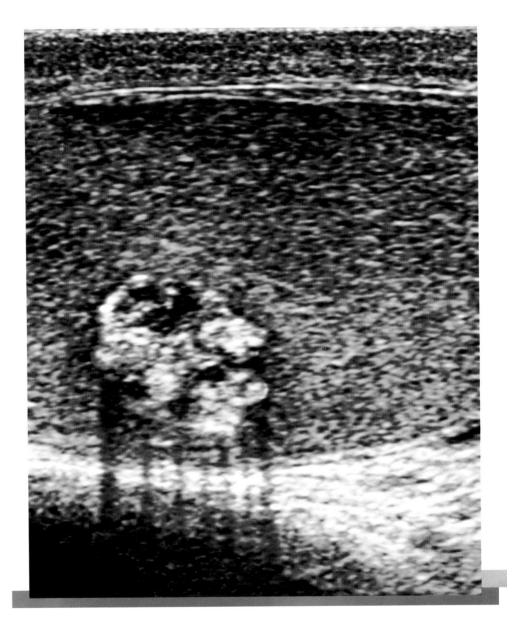

This colored ultrasound scan of a testicle shows a malignant, or cancerous, tumor (colored purple).

body tissues. LDH is released into the blood when tissues suffer damage. High levels of this enzyme may be a sign of cancer but can also result from other diseases. Although blood tests can give doctors clues, other tests are often needed to make a diagnosis.

Scrotal Ultrasound

If any lumps are found in a testicle, a doctor will usually order a scrotal ultrasound to be performed on the patient. An ultrasound is a type of imaging test. An ultrasound produces sound waves that are beamed into the body. The sound waves bounce off the structures of the body, creating echoes that a computer turns into pictures. Tissues of varying densities reflect sound waves differently. In this way, doctors are able to examine images of the bones, organs, and internal tissues.

A scrotal ultrasound yields a picture of the inside of the scrotum. With a scrotal ultrasound, a doctor is able to see the abnormal mass, determine its size and location, and determine if the mass is cancerous or if it is the result of another medical condition (such as an infection). Most testicular cancers will appear as solid (dense) masses on an ultrasound. If the lump appears to be cancerous, a family doctor will refer the patient to a urologist. Urologists specialize in the male and female genitourinary tracts.

Orchiectomy

The only way to know for sure if cancer is present in the body is to look at a sample of the questionable tissue under a microscope. To obtain tissue to examine, a surgeon usually removes the affected testicle through the groin. This procedure is called an inguinal orchiectomy. Biopsies that involve cutting through the scrotum to remove just part of the testicle are not often performed if doctors are worried about testicular cancer because studies have shown that these practices can

Orchiectomy

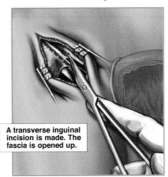

A transverse inguinal incision is made. The fascia is opened up.

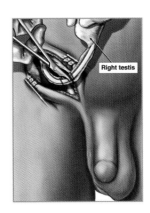

Right testis

Post-operative Condition

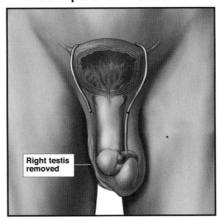

Right testis removed

During an inguinal orchiectomy, surgeons make an incision, which is about 3 inches (7.6 cm) long, in the patient's groin area. The testicle is pulled up through the incision and the spermatic cord is cut. Some patients decide to have a prosthetic testicle inserted into their scrotum after the surgery so that it retains its normal shape.

cause the cancer to spread. Instead, a small incision is made in the lower abdomen. The testicle is then pushed up through the pelvic region and out through the incision. The surgery only takes about forty-five minutes.

The tissue that is removed during an orchiectomy is examined by a pathologist. A pathologist is a doctor who identifies diseases by studying cells and tissues under a microscope. The pathologist can determine which type of testicular cancer it is because each type of testicular cancer looks different under a microscope. With the information that doctors gather from tests, it is also possible to determine the stage of the testicular cancer.

TEN GREAT QUESTIONS
TO ASK YOUR DOCTOR

1. What exactly is cancer?

2. What happens if I get testicular cancer in both testicles?

3. Will losing a testis stop me from producing testosterone and "being a man"?

4. Will having testicular cancer affect my chances of having children someday?

5. What kinds of tests will I need, and do they hurt?

6. What will these tests tell you about my condition?

7. Why did I get testicular cancer?

8. When the time comes for me to have sex, will I be able to?

9. Could my cancer return after treatment?

10. What are the chances that I could die soon from testicular cancer?

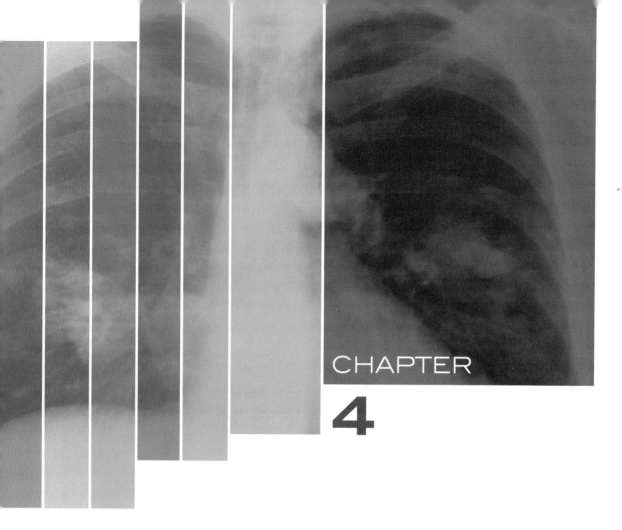

CHAPTER

4

THE STAGES OF TESTICULAR CANCER

If testicular cancer is diagnosed, more tests need to be done to determine if it has spread from the testis to other parts of the body. When testicular cancer spreads, it can do so in one of the following three ways: through tissue by invading the surrounding normal tissue; through the lymph system by traveling through the lymph vessels to other places in the body; or by traveling through the blood to other locations in the body.

The system that is used to describe the location, site, and spread of cancer is called staging. Doctors need to determine what stage testicular

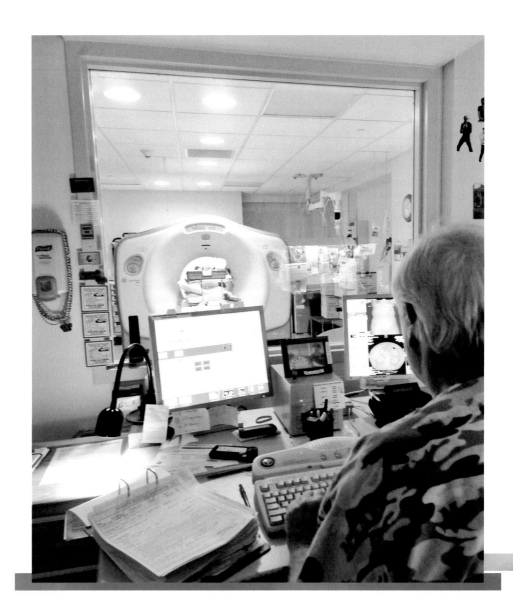

A CT scanner, like the one shown here, uses a computer and an X-ray tube to take many detailed pictures of the part of the body being studied as the X-ray device rotates around the patient. The computer then combines the pictures into a cross-sectional image that shows a two-dimensional slice of the body.

cancer is in so that they can figure out the best way to treat it. To stage the cancer, doctors use blood tests, imaging techniques, and, sometimes, additional surgery. The stages of testicular cancer are described using 0 (for carcinoma in situ) and the Roman numerals I to III. With each higher stage, the cancer described is more severe, or more advanced. Testicular cancer is staged using the TNM system, which was created by the American Joint Committee on Cancer (AJCC). The AJCC is a group of medical organizations that creates systems of classification for cancer that all medical professionals can use.

TNM is an acronym, meaning that each letter represents a different word. "T" stands for "tumor" and represents the size of the tumor and if it has spread to nearby tissues in the testicle. "N" stands for "nodes" and indicates the spread of cancer to the regional (nearby) lymph nodes. The lymph nodes are an important part of a person's immune system. They filter fluids, catching bacteria and viruses. "M" represents the metastasis, or spread, of cancer to distant lymph nodes or other parts of the body. For testicular cancer, there is another level to TNM staging. This level, called "S" for "serum," describes the levels of the tumor markers (like AFP, β-hCG, and LDH discussed in chapter 3) that are produced by some testicular cancers. Additional letters or numbers appear after the T, N, M, and S to indicate increasing severity. For example, T0 means that there is no evidence of a tumor, while T4 indicates that the tumor has grown into the skin surrounding the testes (the scrotum).

TESTICULAR CANCER STAGING TESTS

Some of the tests used to stage testicular cancer are blood tests, imaging tests, and surgery. As described in the previous chapter, the presence of certain tumor markers can help diagnose testicular cancer. The levels of these markers can also help doctors figure out which stage a patient's testicular cancer is. The more of these substances in a man's blood, the more severe, or advanced, his cancer is. Imaging tests are also important when staging testicular cancer. These tests include X-rays, computed tomography (CT) scans, magnetic resonance imaging (MRI) scans, and positron emission tomography (PET) scans.

X-rays are high-energy beams of radiation. This radiation is able to pass through the body. As it does, it creates shadows on a sheet of film. On X-ray film, soft tissue appears dark and bone appears white. Tumors either appear as very dark areas or very light ones, depending on how solid they are. A doctor will perform a chest X-ray on a testicular cancer patient to see if the cancer has spread to the lungs or lymph nodes in the chest. In addition to the X-ray, many doctors may have a CT scan done to better judge if the cancer has spread to the chest.

CT scans use X-rays along with a computer to create thin, clear slices or cross-sectional pictures of the body. A patient lies flat and still on a table while a scanner rotates around it. The scanner shoots thousands of X-ray beams at the area the doctor wants to look at. The X-rays pass through the person and into a detector on the other side. The pictures are displayed on a computer screen. The images clearly show the size, volume, shape, and location of a tumor. Doctors use CT scans to see if testicular cancer has spread to the lymph nodes, liver, lungs, or other organs. Before the scan, a patient may have a dye injected into a vein or be asked to drink a dye that helps outline the abnormal areas in the body. CT scans are painless and take only a few minutes, but they do involve some radiation exposure.

MRI scans use radio waves and very powerful magnets to create a detailed picture of the inside of the body. MRIs are especially useful for examining the brain and spinal cord for evidence of testicular cancer. An MRI is different from other imaging tests because it does not use radiation. The patient lies on a table that moves into a long, cylinder-shaped tube, which is surrounded by a circular magnet. Getting an MRI is painless, but the noise it makes can be very loud. Also, it takes much longer than a CT scan.

NO MORE CLAUSTROPHOBIA

Many people become very claustrophobic during an MRI. Being claustrophobic means that a person is afraid of enclosed or confined places. Some facilities now offer "open" MRIs. An open MRI is an advanced imaging procedure in which the machines have an open design with little or no pounding noise. People who are claustrophobic, too heavy to fit in traditional MRI scanners, or suffering from post-traumatic stress syndrome find the open MRI procedure more comfortable than the closed system.

PET scans are different from CT scans in that they are able to detect active tissues, including cancer. During a PET scan, a radioactive form of sugar is injected into the patient. The body uses sugar for energy. Therefore, sugar is taken up by active cells. Cancer cells are very active and multiply quickly. Consequently, they absorb a lot of the radioactive sugar. During the test, a special camera creates a picture that shows the areas of radioactivity in the body. This image is not as detailed as those given by CT scans or MRIs. However, it provides useful information about the whole body, including the primary tumor and any sites of spreading.

As mentioned in the last chapter, surgery is an essential part of diagnosing, staging, and treating testicular cancer. The stage of testicular cancer can be completely determined only if the testis is surgically removed (inguinal orchiectomy) and examined under a microscope. During the orchiectomy surgery, abdominal and pelvic lymph node dissection is also usually performed to complete the staging. In this procedure, some lymph nodes are removed so that they can be examined for the presence of cancer cells. After looking at the results of all the tests and scans, a doctor will stage a patient's testicular cancer, describing it as being one of the following:

Stage 0 Testicular Cancer: This stage is also called a precancerous condition or carcinoma in situ (CIS). In this stage, there are abnormal cells in the tiny tubules in the testes where sperm is produced. These abnormal cells are confined in the testicle. It makes sense, then, that "in situ" means "in its place" in Latin. It is hard to find testicular cancer in this stage because it generally causes no symptoms. There is often no lump that a doctor can feel. All tumor marker levels are also normal. Sometimes, testicular cancer at this stage is found incidentally when men are undergoing tests for infertility, which is the inability to have children. Researchers have estimated that it may take about five years for carcinoma in situ to progress into invasive cancer.

Stage I Testicular Cancer: About 72 percent of men with testicular cancer have Stage I tumors at the time of diagnosis. Stage I testicular cancer is broken down into three substages: IA, IB, and IS. In stage IA, the cancer is found only in the testicle and the epididymis (the tubules next to the testicles where sperm matures). The cancer may have spread to the inner layer (tunica albuginea) of the double membrane that surrounds the testicle, but it has not spread to the outer layer (tunica vaginalis). The cancer has not yet invaded the blood or lymph vessels, and it has not spread to distant sites. All tumor marker levels are normal. In Stage IB, the cancer has either invaded the blood vessels or lymph nodes within the testicle, has spread to the outer membrane around the testicle (tunica vaginalis), and/or the cancer has invaded the spermatic cord. In Stage IB, all the tumor markers are still normal. In Stage IS, the cancer may

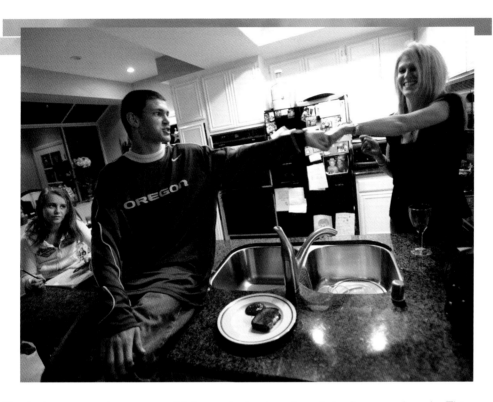

Testicular cancer has a very high survival rate when it is diagnosed early. This young man, shown here with his family, survived cancer and is back to playing with his local basketball club.

be anywhere within the testicle, the spermatic cord, or the scrotum. In addition, one or more of the tumor markers is elevated. In spite of this, the cancer has not yet spread to distant lymph nodes, tissues, or organs. When testicular cancer is Stage I, survival rates are very high—about 99 percent for seminomas and 98 percent for nonseminomas.

Stage II Testicular Cancer: Approximately 19 percent of testicular cancers are in Stage II when they are diagnosed. In this stage, testicular cancer is present in the testes, spermatic cord, or the scrotum and has spread to the regional (close) lymph nodes. There are between five hundred and six hundred lymph nodes throughout the human body. They are clustered in the underarms, neck, chest, groin, and abdomen. In Stage II, testicular cancer has only reached the lymph nodes in the abdomen and groin. It has not spread to more distant lymph nodes or organs. Lower back pain is a sign that testicular cancer has spread to the lymph nodes in the abdomen.

Stage II is divided into substages IIA, IIB, and IIC, depending on how big the lymph nodes have become. The bigger the lymph node, the more cancer it contains. Therefore, a bigger lymph node is considered to be a sign that the cancer is more advanced. In Stage II testicular cancer, serum tumor marker levels are normal or slightly elevated. Stage II testicular cancer has a survival rate of about 95 percent for both seminomas and nonseminomas.

Stage III Testicular Cancer: About 9 percent of testicular cancer is Stage III, which is divided into Stages IIIA, IIIB, and IIIC. Stage IIIA testicular cancer has spread to distant lymph nodes (such as those in the chest or above the collarbone) or to the lungs. Serum markers are at normal levels or are slightly elevated. In Stage IIIB, the cancer has spread to any lymph nodes and/or the lungs but not to any other organs. The blood markers are substantially raised. In Stage IIIC, the serum marker levels are extremely elevated, and the cancer has spread to the lymph nodes and/or at least one organ other than the lungs. Even when testicular cancer spreads to other organs, only about one out of four men experiences obvious symptoms. If the testicular cancer has spread to the lungs, a man may have trouble breathing, may cough, or may have chest pain. He may even cough up blood. If the cancer has spread to the liver, he may experience

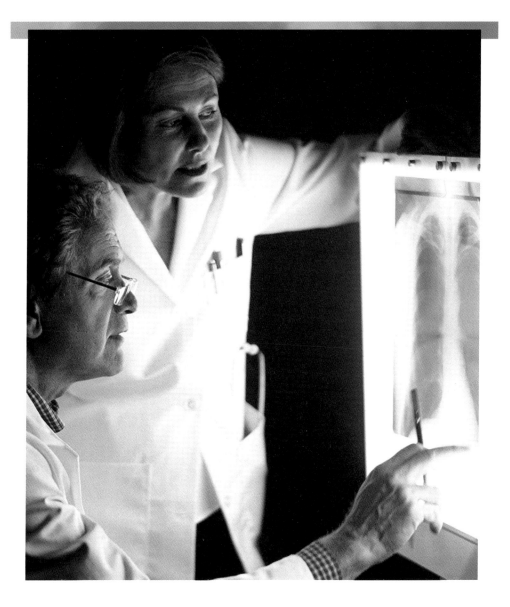

Chest X-rays, like this one, are often used to determine whether testicular cancer has spread to the lungs. When testicular cancer has spread to distant organs, such as the liver, brain, or lungs, it is classified as Stage III testicular cancer.

abdominal pain. If it spreads to the brain, he may have headaches. However, it is rare for testicular cancer to metastasize to the brain. A man with Stage III seminoma still has a survival rate of about 90 percent. However, the survival rate for those with Stage III nonseminoma drops to about 76 percent.

Relapsed Testicular Cancer

Relapsed testicular cancer is cancer that appears again after it has been in remission (all visible signs of the tumor have been eliminated). Testicular cancer could even recur years after the initial cancer is detected. The cancer may return in the same location as the original, or it may appear in a different part of the body. This cancer may be resistant to some forms of treatment, such as some chemotherapy medicines.

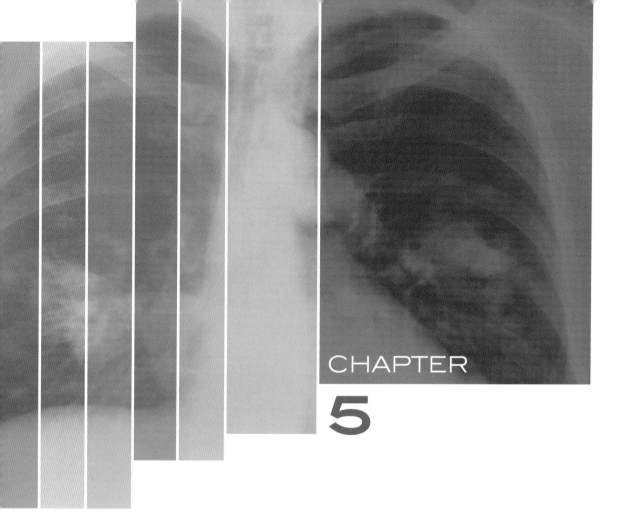

TREATING TESTICULAR CANCER TODAY AND IN THE FUTURE

The results of the staging process will help determine a man's treatment options. The three main treatment options for testicular cancer are surgery, radiation therapy, and chemotherapy. Doctors usually use a combination of these treatments. Surgery is the main treatment for testicular cancer. It is one of the first procedures done because it is also part of the diagnosis and staging. If a patient has Stage I testicular

Imaging equipment, like this multipurpose gamma camera (also known as noninvasive MRI), can be used to diagnose and stage testicular cancer and to monitor a patient after his treatment. Active surveillance of testicular cancer patients has become an increasingly popular option. Improved imaging tools are constantly being created for the purpose of monitoring the progression of the disease.

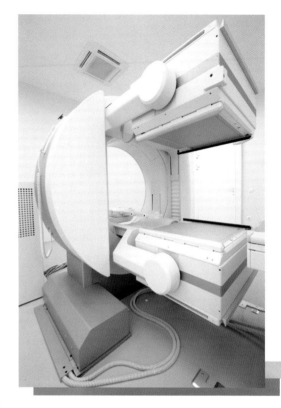

cancer, surgical removal of the testis may be the only needed treatment. Following surgery, patients in Stage I will still undergo surveillance, meaning that the patient is regularly monitored by his doctor for any signs of the cancer's return. Surveillance includes physical examination, blood tests, and/or imaging studies. Following an orchiectomy, a Stage I testicular cancer patient may also be given the option of chemotherapy or radiation, depending on the type of testicular cancer.

RADIATION THERAPY

Radiation therapy uses high-energy rays to kill cancer cells. It works by damaging the DNA in the cells, causing them to die. Cancer cells are more likely to be affected by radiation because most divide more rapidly than healthy cells. However, some healthy cells are also destroyed during radiation therapy. Radiation therapy itself is painless, although it can cause side effects, depending on the site being radiated and the length of the treatment. The most common side effects are tiredness, nausea, diarrhea, dry skin, and loss of appetite. Radiation therapy is used after surgery to prevent the cancer from coming back. It is also used to treat the spread of cancer cells to the lymph nodes. Seminomas are very sensitive to radiation therapy, and many intermediate- and late-stage seminomas are treated with radiation. Nonseminomas, however, do not respond as well to radiation therapy, so they are treated with surgery and chemotherapy if indicated.

CHEMOTHERAPY

Chemotherapy, often called "chemo," is a type of treatment that uses chemicals or drugs to kill cancer cells. These drugs are injected into the body or given orally (by mouth). Chemotherapy destroys cancer cells throughout the body. This is unlike radiation therapy, which concentrates treatment on a specific area. Chemotherapy is routinely used if the cancer has spread to the lymph nodes or other organs. Chemotherapy is also used to treat relapsed testicular cancer.

The drugs used in chemotherapy work by disrupting rapidly dividing cells, like cancer cells. However, chemotherapy also affects other rapidly dividing healthy cells in the body. Hair follicles and the cells lining the digestive tract divide rapidly. Therefore, these cells can be affected by chemotherapy. This explains the hair loss, upset stomach, and mouth sores associated with some chemotherapy. Some chemotherapy drugs (but not all) can cause infertility because sperm and egg cells are very sensitive to these drugs. Some chemotherapy drugs cause low blood counts, which can result in tiredness, bleeding, and risk of infection. The most common drugs used to treat testicular

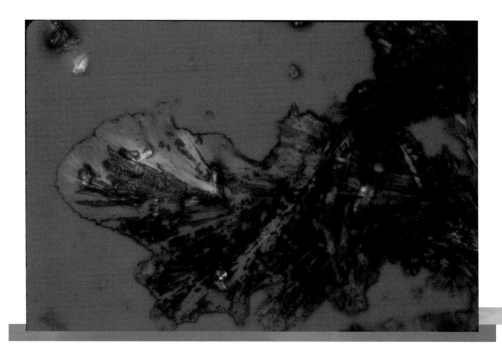

This image shows cisplatin crystals. This chemotherapy drug is usually used in combination with the drugs etoposide and bleomycin. When they are all given together, the therapy is known as BEP.

cancer are bleomycin, etoposide, and cisplatin (in combination they are called BEP). Side effects of these three specific drugs include breathing difficulty, liver problems, allergic reactions, hearing loss, nerve problems, and kidney problems. Other chemotherapy agents may be used for more aggressive types or recurrent cancers.

AFTER TREATMENT

The two functions of the testes are to produce male hormones and produce sperm. Depending on the type of treatment that a man receives for his testicular cancer, one or both of these functions may be affected. Infertility is a major consequence of testicular cancer treatment. Most of the drugs that are used during chemotherapy will damage the testicle's ability to produce sperm, at least temporarily. Though it is usually reversible, this damage is sometimes permanent. Because it is difficult to predict if the condition will be permanent, sperm cryopreservation (sperm banking) is recommended before a patient's cancer treatment begins. Most men are able to father children after an orchiectomy in which just one testicle is removed. However, if both testicles are to be removed, a man wanting to have children in the future should ask about the process of cryopreservation. It's also important for men getting chemotherapy to practice birth control, like using condoms during sex, because these drugs can affect sperm and might cause birth defects in a developing embryo.

LAWRENCE H. EINHORN, DISTINGUISHED PROFESSOR AND LANCE ARMSTRONG FOUNDATION PROFESSOR OF ONCOLOGY

Lawrence H. Einhorn, an oncologist (a doctor who studies tumors) at the Indiana University School of Medicine in Indianapolis, is best known for the chemotherapy regimen that he developed in 1974. This treatment included the drug cisplatin, which was fairly new at the time. Einhorn's research gave testicular cancer the high cure rate that it has today. He treated his most famous patient, Lance Armstrong, in 1996. Einhorn joined Armstrong in helping to educate men about the disease, and he became the first Lance Armstrong Foundation Professor of Oncology in 2006. Einhorn continues to contribute valuable findings in the area of testicular cancer research.

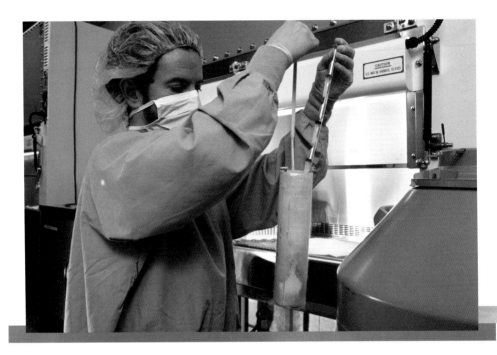

Sperm can be frozen and stored in facilities, such as this one, for future use. The sperm can be frozen indefinitely and then thawed when a patient would like to try to achieve pregnancy with his mate.

Recent studies have shown that about 15 percent of male cancer survivors in general experience testosterone deficiency (shortage) as a late side effect of chemotherapy or radiation therapy. These men complain of reduced energy levels and impaired sexual function. Removing just one testis does not usually affect a man's production of testosterone. The remaining testis is generally able to produce normal levels of the hormone. When both testes have been removed, however, a man will no longer be able to produce testosterone. Without testosterone, a man may experience loss of sexual desire, impotence (the inability to obtain an erection) hot flashes, mood swings, or depression. However, medical advances have made it easy to "replace" the testosterone in the body. There are different hormone replacement options for men today. A man can use daily gel or cream applications, wear a patch, or receive injections.

What the Future Holds

Due to advances in treatment, testicular cancer is one of the most curable forms of cancer today. However, doctors and scientists are still working to discover new approaches to treatment, new information about its causes, and ways to increase the quality of life for cancer survivors. Cancer organizations conduct clinical trials to see how well new medical approaches work in people. The studies are used to find better ways to prevent, diagnose, and treat testicular cancer. A new type of treatment being tested in clinical trials is a high-dose chemotherapy with a stem cell transplant "rescue" from the patient. Although testicular cancers respond well to chemotherapy, not all are cured. Higher doses of chemotherapy would be more effective, but they would damage the bone marrow to such a degree that it could not adequately make new blood cells. For a stem cell transplant, doctors collect stem cells from the bloodstream of a person prior to giving chemotherapy and freeze the cells. These blood-forming stem cells can then be transplanted back to the patient after the treatment is over, thereby "rescuing" them from the toxic effects of the high-dose chemotherapy.

Better ways to deliver radiation therapy are also being investigated. The radiation exposure from testicular cancer treatment has sometimes been shown to increase a man's risk of developing other malignancies, such as leukemia (cancer of the white blood cells). Researchers are, therefore, always looking for new methods to deliver radiation that minimize the exposure to healthy tissues. New techniques have also emerged, such as immunotherapy, which causes the body's own natural defenses (immune system) to attack the testicular cancer or lessen the side effects of other treatments.

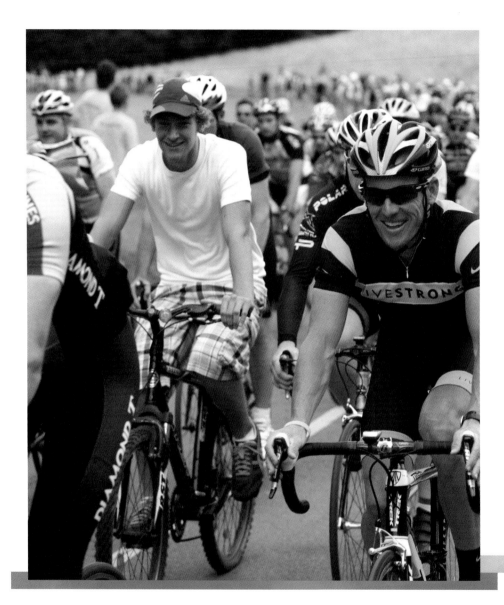

Lance Armstrong (far right), U.S. professional cyclist, is shown riding around Phoenix Park in Dublin, Ireland, with Irish cycling fans. Armstrong continues to be a symbol of hope and inspiration for the fight against testicular cancer.

Researchers are always looking for new risk factors for testicular cancer. Doctors at the Fred Hutchinson Cancer Research Center in Seattle, Washington, have just recently discovered a link between the disease and marijuana use. Studies have also suggested that there may be a link to obesity as well. In an attempt to find the genes involved in causing testicular cancer, clinical researchers from fourteen different countries have come together to form the International Testicular Cancer Linkage Consortium (ITCLC). Scientists have identified several genes whose mutations lead to an increased risk of developing testicular cancer. However, they are still seeking to identify more. As more genes are linked to the development of testicular cancer, doctors will be able to diagnose the disease earlier and to provide improved treatment.

Even though there is much more to be learned in the field of cancer, medical researchers have come a long way since Aulus Cornelius Celsus wrote *De medicina octo libri*. People no longer have to have a grim view of cancer. In 2000, Lance Armstrong launched the Cycle of Hope, a national cancer education campaign for people who have cancer or who are at risk for developing it. "I ignored my symptoms until it was almost too late," Armstrong said. "I am dedicated to the Cycle of Hope campaign because I want to help others break out of their cycle of misunderstanding and fear and empower themselves through the Cycle of Hope."

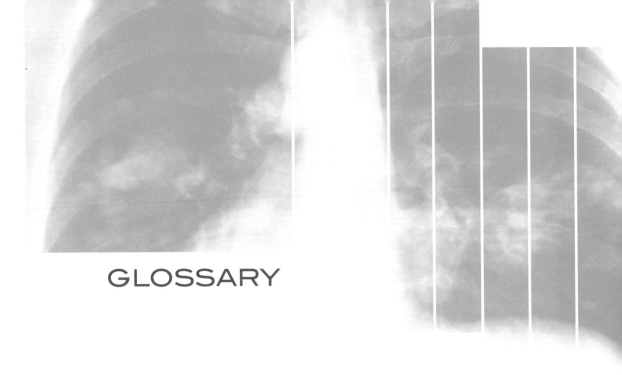

GLOSSARY

abdomen The area of the body that contains the intestines, stomach, liver, pancreas, kidneys, and other organs.

abnormal Not normal; different from the usual condition.

antibiotic A substance that is able to kill bacteria.

benign A tumor that is not likely to spread.

bloodstream The flow of blood around the body.

cancer A malignant, invasive tumor or growth.

cauterize To burn tissue of a wound by applying a heated instrument to it so that the wound will not become infected.

cell The basic unit of living organisms.

cell division A process by which a cell divides to form two new cells.

chemical reaction A change in which one kind of matter is turned into another kind of matter.

congenital Present at birth.

density Compactness.

DNA (deoxyribonucleic acid) The genetic information of organisms that makes up chromosomes and is located in the nucleus of a cell.

electrolysis The process in which electricity is passed through a liquid between electrodes.

endocrine system The glands of the body that release hormones to direct the body's processes.

enzyme A molecule that speeds up a chemical reaction.

immune system The system of the body that recognizes and fights disease.

incidence Occurrence.

infertility The condition in which a person is unable to have children.

invasive cancer A cancer that tends to spread from one place to another in the body.

malignant A tumor that is likely to grow large and spread.

metastasis The spread of a tumor from one part of the body to other parts.

nonseminoma A type of testicular cancer arising from germ cells.

organ An independent part of the body that serves a specific function.

papyrus An ancient form of paper made from the papyrus plant, which grows along the Nile River.

pelvis The basin-shaped ring of hip bones near the base of the spine to which the legs are attached.

pure Not mixed.

recurrent Returning or happening repeatedly.

seminoma The most common kind of testicular cancer arising from germ cells.

side effect An unintended effect or problem caused by treatment.

testis The male reproductive gland (gonad); the plural form of testis is testes.

tissue A group of cells in an organism.

tumor An abnormal mass of tissue.

urologist A doctor who specializes in the urinary tract of males and females and the male reproductive organs.

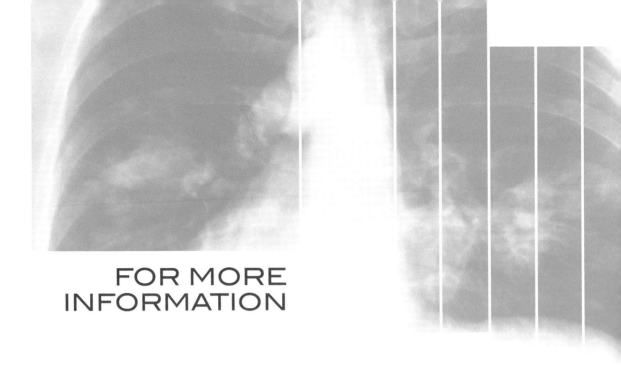

FOR MORE INFORMATION

American Cancer Society (ACS)
1599 Clifton Road NE
Atlanta, GA 30329-4251
(800) 227-2345
Web site: http://www.cancer.org
The ACS is a nationwide health organization dedicated to cancer research and education and patient services.

American Society of Clinical Oncology (ASCO)
1900 Duke Street, Suite 200
Alexandria, VA 22314
(703) 299-0150
Web site: http://www.asco.org
The ASCO is a nonprofit organization with the goal of improving cancer care and prevention.

Cancer Research Institute (CRI)
One Exchange Plaza

55 Broadway, Suite 1802
New York, NY 10006
(800) 99CANCER (992-2623)
Web site: http://www.cancerresearch.org
The CRI supports and coordinates laboratory and clinical efforts that
will lead to the immunological treatment, control, and prevention
of cancer.

CureSearch
Children's Oncology Group
Research Operations Center
440 East Huntington Drive, Suite 400
Arcadia, CA 91006-3776
(800) 458-6223
Web site: http://www.curesearch.org/for_parents_and_families
CureSearch provides information about clinical trials for pediatric
oncology patients.

Kids Count, Too
American Cancer Society
15999 Clifton Road NE
Atlanta, GA 30329
(800) ACS-2345 (227-2345)
Web site: http://www.cancer.org
This organization provides information about surviving cancer of any
kind, including testicular cancer. There is a support group, Look
Good…Feel Better for Teens, for cancer patients between the ages
of thirteen and seventeen (and a Web site, www.2bme.org).

Livestrong Lance Armstrong Foundation
2201 East Sixth Street

Austin, TX 78702

(866) 673-7205

Web site: http://www.livestrong.org

Livestrong funds important projects to advance the field of cancer survivor research and improve the quality of life for cancer survivors.

National Cancer Institute

6116 Executive Boulevard, Room 3036A

Bethesda, MD 20892

(800) 4-CANCER (422-6237)

Web site: http://www.cancer.gov

The National Cancer Institute is a component of the National Institutes of Health. It is dedicated to the prevention, diagnosis, and treatment of cancer.

Planned Parenthood Federation of America, Inc. (PPFA)

434 West Thirty-third Street

New York, NY 10001

(800) 230-7526

Web site: http://www.plannedparenthood.org

The PPFA offers information on how to do testicular self-exams, the signs and symptoms of problems, and the treatment of testicular cancer.

Prevent Cancer Foundation

1600 Duke Street, Suite 500

Alexandria, VA 22314

(800) 227-2732

Web site: http://www.preventcancer.org

The foundation provides easy-to-understand information about testicular cancer and suggests ways to lower cancer risk

Testicular Cancer Resource Center
Web site: http://tcrc.acor.org
This patient-oriented Web site is written in plain language for young
    men and adults. It includes links to a list of testicular cancer experts
    that your doctor can consult, helpful hints, humor, alternative treat-
    ments, and more than eighty personal stories. It offers private,
    individual e-mail support.

WEB SITES

Due to the changing nature of Internet links, Rosen Publishing has
developed an online list of Web sites related to the subject of this book.
This site is updated regularly. Please use this link to access the list:

http://www.rosenlinks.com/cms/test

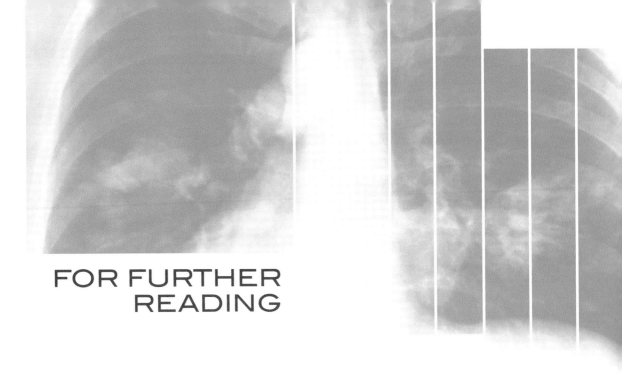

FOR FURTHER READING

Armentrout, David, and Patricia Armentrout. *Lance Armstrong (Discover the Life of a Sports Star)*. New York, NY: Rourke Publishing, 2003.

Armstrong, Lance. *Livestrong*. Portland, OR: Broadway Books, 2005.

Banks, Ian. *Haynes Owners Workshop Manual—Cancer Any Age, Any Time*. Somerset, England: J. H. Haynes and Company, Ltd., 2004.

Bozzone, Donna. *Cancer Genetics* (The Biology of Cancer). New York, NY: Chelsea House, 2007.

Bozzone, Donna. *Causes of Cancer* (The Biology of Cancer). New York, NY: Chelsea House, 2010.

Caldwell, Wilma R., ed. *Cancer Information for Teens: Health Tips About Cancer Awareness, Prevention, Diagnosis, and Treatment* (Teen Health Series). Detroit, MI: Omnigraphics, 2004.

Garcia, Kimberly. *Lance Armstrong*. Hockessin, DE: Mitchell Lane Publishers, 2005.

Gillie, Oliver. *Just the Facts: Cancer*. Chicago, IL: Heinemann Library, 2004.

Hecht, Alan, and David Triggle. *Understanding Drugs! Cancer Treatment Drugs*. New York, NY: Chelsea House, 2010.

Johanson, Paula. *Frequently Asked Questions About Testicular Cancer* (FAQ: Teen Life). New York, NY: Rosen Publishing Group, 2008

Kenny, Paraic. *Stages of Cancer Development* (The Biology of Cancer). New York, NY: Chelsea House, 2007.

McKinnell, Robert Gilmore. *Prevention of Cancer* (The Biology of Cancer). New York, NY: Chelsea House, 2008.

Panno, Joseph. *The Role of Genes, Lifestyle, and Environment* (New Biology). New York, NY: Facts On File, 2004.

Priestman, Terry. *The Cancer Survivor's Handbook*. London, England: Sheldon Press, 2009.

Priestman, Terry. *Coping with Chemotherapy*. London, England: Sheldon Press, 2005.

Priestman, Terry. *Coping with Radiotherapy*. London, England: Sheldon Press, 2007.

Royston, Angela. *Cancer*. Chicago, IL: Heinemann Library, 2006.

Silverstein, Alvin, et al. *Cancer: Conquering a Deadly Disease*. New York, NY: Twenty-First Century Books, 2004.

Verville, Kathleen. *Testicular Cancer*. New York, NY: Facts On File, 2009.

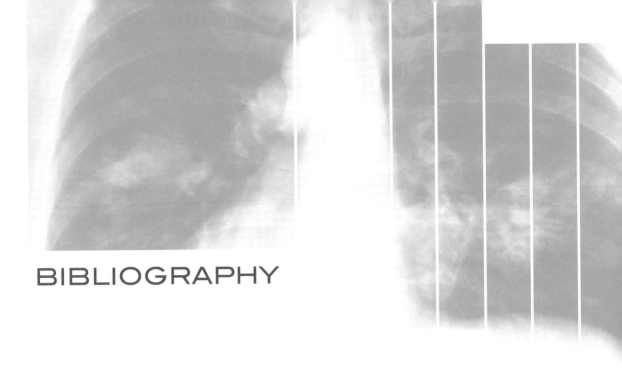

BIBLIOGRAPHY

Advameg. "Aulus Cornelius Celsus Biography (c. 25 BCE–c. 50 CE)." Retrieved March 5, 2010 (http://www.faqs.org/health/bios/65/Aulus-Cornelius-Celsus.html).

American Association for Clinical Chemistry. "Testicular Cancer." March 6, 2010. Retrieved March 12, 2010 (http://www.labtestsonline.org/understanding/conditions/testicular.html).

American Cancer Society. "Detailed Guide: Testicular Cancer." August 3, 2009. Retrieved March 14, 2010 (http://www.cancer.org/docroot/CRI/content/CRI_2_4_1X_What_is_testicular_cancer_41.asp).

American Society of Clinical Oncology. "Testicular Cancer." March 2009. Retrieved March 13, 2010 (http://www.cancer.net/patient/Cancer+Types/Testicular+Cancer).

Benowitz, Steven I. *Cancer*. Berkeley Heights, NJ: Enslow Publishers, 1999.

Chemical Heritage Foundation. "Methods of Treatment: Cisplatin: The Platinum Standard." 2001. Retrieved March 14, 2010 (http://www.chemheritage.org/EducationalServices/pharm/chemo/readings/cisplat.htm).

Ingraham, J. L., and C. A. Ingraham. *Introduction to Microbiology*. 3rd ed. Pacific Grove, CA: Brooks/Cole–Thomson Learning, 2004.

James Buchanan Brady Urological Institute. "Testicular Cancer." March 16, 2010. Retrieved March 17, 2010 (http://urology.jhu.edu/testis/cancer.php?var=overview.php).

Lawton, Sandra Augustyn. *Sexual Health Information for Teens*. Detroit, MI: Omnigraphics, 2008.

Medscape. "Lance Armstrong Launches Cycle of Hope Cancer Campaign." February 14, 2000. Retrieved March 15, 2010 (http://www.medscape.com/viewarticle/411558).

Morrow, Alina. "Testicular Cancer." May 4, 2009. Retrieved on March 13, 2010 (http://www.omnimedicalsearch.com/conditions-diseases/testicular-cancer-overview.html).

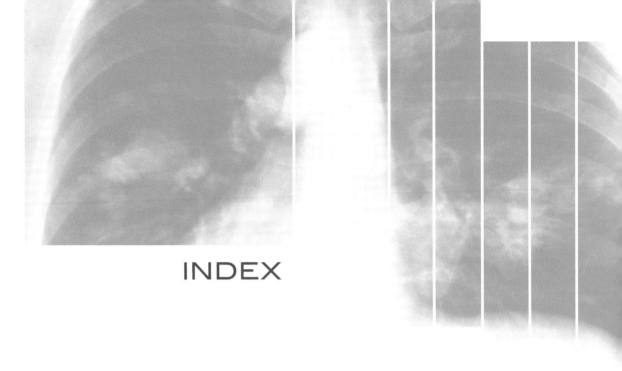

INDEX

ABOUT THE AUTHOR

Heather Hasan graduated summa cum laude from East Stroudsburg University with a dual major in chemistry and biochemistry. She has also written books about cervical cancer and bone cancer. She currently lives in Durham, North Carolina, with her husband, Omar, their sons, Samuel and Matthew, and their daughter, Sarah Elizabeth.

PHOTO CREDITS

Cover, p. 1 © Science Photo Library/CMSP; cover (top), pp. 4–5 (bottom) Punchstock; back cover pp. 3, 7, 16, 23, 33, 43, 46, 52, 54, 58, 60, 62 National Cancer Institute; p. 5 Lynn Johnson/Sports Illustrated/Getty Images; p. 9 Nucleus Medical Art, Inc./Getty Images; p. 11 MedImage/Photo Researchers, Inc.; p. 14 Yorgos Nikas/ Stone/Getty Images; p. 18 Comstock/Thinkstock; pp. 19, 30 Medical Animation Copyright © 2010 Nucleus Medical Media, All rights reserved. www.nucleusinc.com; p. 20 BananaStock/Thinkstock; p. 24 Marvin Joseph/The Washington Post/Getty Images; p. 28 Du Cane Medical Imaging, Ltd./Photo Researchers, Inc.; p. 34 John Guillemin/Bloomberg/Getty Images; p. 39 © The Orange County Register/ZUMA Press; p. 41 Digital Vision/Thinkstock; p. 44 © www.istockphoto.com/zilli; p. 48 Jon Meyer/CMSP; p. 50 Peter Muhly/AFP/Getty Images.

Designer: Evelyn Horovicz; Editor: Kathy Kuhtz Campbell;
Photo Researcher: Amy Feinberg